Table of Contents

Diabetes mellitus refers to a group of diseases that affect how the body uses blood sugar (glucose). Glucose is an important source of energy for the cells that make up the muscles and tissues. It's also the brain's main source of fuel.

The main cause of diabetes varies by type. But no matter what type of diabetes you have, it can lead to excess sugar in the blood. Too much sugar in the blood can lead to serious health problems.

Chronic diabetes conditions include type 1 diabetes and type 2 diabetes. Potentially reversible diabetes conditions include prediabetes and gestational diabetes. Prediabetes happens when blood sugar levels are higher than normal. But the blood sugar levels aren't high enough to be called diabetes. And prediabetes can lead to diabetes unless steps are taken to prevent it. Gestational diabetes happens during pregnancy. But it may go away after the baby is born.

BREAKFAST

1. Muffins with Spinach & Feta

Prep Time: 15 Minutes

Cook Time: 25 Minutes

Servings: 4

Ingredients

- 4 cups spinach, washed
- 2 scallions, thinly chopped
- 1 leek, chopped
- 4oz/110g feta cheese
- 1/2 cup and 2 tbsp quick oats
- 3 eggs
- 1 heaping tbsp yogurt
- 3 tbsp olive oil or 2 heaping tbsp butter, room temp
- Pinch of baking soda

Instructions

1. Saute the leeks and scallions with some olive oil for 1-2 minutes. Add spinach and cover for 6-7 minutes until the spinach is wilted. Then stir without a lid for 2 more minutes and turn the heat off.
2. Preheat the oven to 180C or 350F.
3. Add eggs, olive oil, crumbled feta, yogurt, baking soda and oats to a bowl and blend using an immersion blender.
4. Add in the cooked cooled-off spinach.
5. Line a muffin pan with parchment paper muffin liners (other varieties can make releasing the baked muffins harder).
6. Fill muffin cups with the mixture and bake for about 25 minutes or until firm to the touch and golden brown.
7. Let cool off. If stuck to the pan - use a knife and carefully work your way around the edges to release the muffins. Enjoy!

Prep Time: 10 Minutes

Cook Time: 30 Minutes

Servings: 6

Ingredients

Apples:

- 6 sweet apples
- 1 tbsp cinnamon
- pinch of salt
- 2 tsp coconut oil

Crumble:

- 2/3 cup oats
- 2/3 cup pecans
- 1 tbsp coconut oil
- 2 tsp honey

Instructions

1. Chop the apples and saute them in a pan with the rest
   of the ingredients at medium-high. I covered the pan
   for 2-3 minutes.
2. Preheat your oven to 180C/350F.
3. Put all crumble ingredients into your food processor
   (blender or immersion blender might work too), add a
   splash of water (about 1 tbsp), and process until you
   get a crumbly mixture that sticks together.
4. Use a small baking pan, oil the surface or add
   parchment paper and spread the apples. Then squeeze
   the crumble mixture to form bigger pieces of crumble
   and spread these over the apples.
5. Bake for 15-20 minutes or until the crumble is golden
   brown.
6. Let cool off a little bit and enjoy with some
   milk/yogurt for breakfast or ice cream for dessert.

Prep Time: 10 Minutes

Cook Time: 20 Minutes

Servings: 3

Ingredients

- 3 large burrito size flour tortillas
- 1 cup black refried beans (or regular refried beans)
- 3 eggs
- 2 tablespoons butter
- Salt and pepper to taste
- 1 and ½ cup Mexican blend shredded cheese
- Sour cream, guacamole, and/or hot sauce, for serving

Instructions

1. On a large size non-stick skillet, melt 1 tablespoon of butter and scramble 3 eggs. Season with salt and pepper. Set the eggs aside. We will use the same pan to cook the quesadilla.
2. Make a halfway cut on large flour tortillas from the center to the edge (cut a line from the center of the

tortilla to the bottom edge). Gently fold the tortilla in 3 so it will leave folding marks to guide us where to put the fillings.

3. On the first area (the left side from the cut), spread ⅓ cup of refried beans evenly. Add the scrambled egg on top. Press gently on the eggs so they will stick to the refried bean.

4. On the rest of the area (⅔ of the tortilla), spread ½ cup of the cheese evenly.

5. Lift the side with the beans and eggs and fold it towards the second area. And fold once more to make the 3 layers.

6. Set it aside and repeat with the rest of the tortillas to make 3 quesadillas.

7. Heat the pan with ⅓ tablespoon of butter on medium heat. Add the assembled quesadilla to the pan. Cook until it is golden brown, about 2 to 4 minutes. Carefully flip the quesadilla and cook the other side for a couple more minutes.

8. Serve with sour cream, guacamole, and/or hot sauce.

Prep Time: 10 Minutes

Cook Time: 25 Minutes

Servings: 2

Ingredients

For smoked paprika garlic aioli:

- ¼ cup mayo
- 1 clove garlic, grated using a micro grater
- 2 teaspoons fresh lemon juice
- ¼ teaspoon smoked paprika
- Salt and pepper to taste

For tater tot breakfast hash (breakfast totchos):

- Half bag of frozen tater tots (about 14 to 16 ounces)
- 1 tablespoon oil, divided
- 2 eggs
- ⅓ cup caramelized onion
- 1 avocado, cut into bite-size pieces
- ⅓ cup red bell pepper (half of a pepper), sliced thinly
- salt and pepper to taste

Instructions

1. For smoked paprika garlic aioli (Make this first)
2. Mix all ingredients in a small bowl.
3. Keep in the fridge for at least 30 minutes to develop its flavor. It should keep in the fridge for up to 10 days.
4. For tater tot breakfast hash (breakfast totchos)
5. Cook the tater tots in the air fryer at 400F for 12 minutes. Shake and continue to cook for additional 3 more minutes.
6. While you are cooking tater tots, fry 2 eggs. Season with salt and pepper. Take the egg out of the pan once it is cooked to your liking.
7. On the same pan, add 1 teaspoon of oil and add the sliced red bell pepper. Season with salt and pepper. Cook for 2 to 3 minutes with frequent stirring. Set it aside.
8. Once the tater tot is done, assemble the breakfast hash. Add the tater tots to the dish that you are serving. Add the caramelized onion and cooked pepper on top. Place the avocado and cooked egg on top. Drizzle with aioli.

Prep Time: 10 Minutes

Cook Time: 1hrs 25 Minutes

Servings: 10

Ingredients

- 2-3 bananas, ripe, approx 1 1/4 cups mashed
- 1 banana, fresh
- 2 cups almond flour
- 1/2 cup tapioca flour
- 1 tsp baking soda
- 1 tsp ground cinnamon
- 1/4 tsp salt
- 2 eggs, large
- 1/4 cup butter, or coconut oil, melted
- 1/4 cup honey
- 1 tsp vanilla extract
- Additional Butter Or Coconut Oil Is Needed To Grease The Loaf Pan

Instructions

1. Preheat the oven to 350 degrees fahrenheit.

2. Use butter or coconut oil to grease the inside of a loaf pan (8.5 x 4.5 inch) and set aside.

3. Mash the bananas with a fork in a mixing bowl. Add the remaining ingredients, then use a hand mixer to blend everything together for 30 seconds. Pour the batter into the loaf pan

4. Peel and slice the fresh banana in half lengthwise, then place it on top of the batter.

5. Cook the banana bread for 50-60 minutes. If the top gets too golden, you can cover with a piece of aluminum foil. Use a toothpick to test that the banana bread is cooked through.

6. Remove the banana bread and let it cool for 5 minutes in the loaf pan. Then slice it up and enjoy.

Prep Time: 15 Minutes

Cook Time: 1hrs 20 Minutes

Servings: 12

Ingredients

- 1 pound sweet potato, peeled and diced into 1/2" cubes
- 1 tablespoon olive oil
- 1/4 teaspoon garlic powder
- 1/4 teaspoon paprika
- 1/4 teaspoon cumin
- salt and pepper
- 8 ounces bacon
- 1 pound breakfast sausage, mild, medium or spicy, your choice
- 1/2 large onion, diced
- 1 green bell pepper, deseeded and diced
- 2 cloves garlic, minced
- 12 large eggs
- 1/3 cup milk, dairy or dairy-free
- optional: shredded cheese and green onion for garnish

Instructions

1. Preheat your oven to 400F/200C and get a 9×13 casserole pan out. On one baking sheet pan, toss the diced sweet potato with olive oil, garlic powder, paprika, cumin, salt, and pepper. Set aside.

2. Sweet potatoes on a baking sheet.

3. On another sheet pan, add slices of bacon. Then place both the sweet potato and bacon in the oven and cook for 18-20 minutes, or until the bacon is done. The bacon will be done first, so keep an eye on it and remove it from the oven when it's done, and place on paper towels to dry. Stir the sweet potato and continue cooking it for another 15 minutes.

4. Bacon and sweet potatoes on baking sheets.

5. While the sweet potato is cooking, cook the breakfast sausage in a pan on medium high heat. Once it's browned, remove it with a slotted spoon and place it in the casserole pan.

6. Browning breakfast sausage in a pan.

7. Drain off all but a tablespoon of grease from the pan, then saute the onion and bell pepper for 4-5 minutes. Add the minced garlic and saute another 30 seconds. Transfer the onion and bell pepper to the casserole pan.

8. Sauteeing bell pepper and onion for a loaded breakfast casserole.

9. Remove the sweet potato from the oven and add it to the casserole pan, with the crumbled bacon, onion, and bell pepper. If you'd like to add cheese, you can add it to the casserole pan now.

10. Breakfast casserole ingredients in a casserole dish.

11. Stir all of the ingredients in the casserole pan together. Feel free to season with more salt and pepper.

12. Stir ingredients in a pan for a loaded breakfast casserole.

13. In a mixing bowl, stir the eggs with the milk.

14. Whisking egg mixture for a loaded breakfast casserole.

15. Pour the egg mixture on top of the meat and vegetables. Cook for 25-30 minutes, or until the center is cooked through and the edges are slightly golden. You can test the center with a toothpick.

16. Pouring egg mixture into a pan for a loaded breakfast casserole.

17. If you'd like, garnish the breakfast casserole with green onion, or herbs. Then serve warm with sliced avocado, toast, or a side salad.

Prep Time: 15 Minutes

Cook Time: 40 Minutes

Servings: 8

Ingredients

- 10 large eggs
- ½ cup yogurt, or dairy-free yogurt
- 2 tablespoons olive oil
- 1 leek, white and light green parts chopped
- ½ pound thin asparagus, trimmed and cut into 1/2-inch pieces
- 1 cup frozen peas
- 1 cup (packed) baby spinach
- salt and pepper, to taste
- 4 ounces goat cheese, or feta/other cheese
- Optional garnish: fresh dill, and parsley

Instructions

1. Preheat the oven to 400F/200C. Heat the oil in a 10-inch oven-safe skillet over medium heat. Add the leek and saute for 3-4 minutes.
2. Then add the asparagus and saute another 1-2 minutes.
3. Sauteeing leeks and asparagus for spring vegetable frittata
4. Then add the frozen peas, baby spinach, salt and pepper, and saute another 1-2 minutes, or until the spinach is wilted. Remove 1/3 of the vegetables to a plate (optional, but it makes for a prettier frittata), and make sure the remaining half of vegetables is evenly spread out.
5. Sauteeing vegetable for spring vegetable frittata.
6. In a large bowl, whisk the eggs, yogurt, salt and pepper. Pour the eggs over the half of the vegetables in the pan. Cook on the stove for 2-3 minutes.
7. Add the remaining vegetables on top, then dollop with the goat cheese. Transfer to the oven and cook for 15-20 minutes, or until the eggs are set.
8. Cooking eggs with vegetables in a pan for a spring frittata
9. Garnish with additional herbs before serving.

Prep Time: 15 Minutes

Cook Time: 25 Minutes

Servings: 4

Ingredients

- 1 pound Yukon gold potatoes, about 2 small or one large
- 2 tablespoons olive oil
- 2 green onions, sliced
- 2 garlic cloves, minced
- 1 1/2 cups cooked turkey, small diced
- 1/2 cup dried cranberries
- 1 1/2 teaspoons finely chopped fresh thyme, or 1/2 teaspoon dried thyme
- salt and pepper, to taste
- Optional: eggs, top with poached eggs or soft boiled eggs

Instructions

1. Peel and dice the potatoes into a small 1/2" dice.

2. Peeling and dicing the potatoes.

3. Add the potatoes to a pot and cover with cold water. Bring the water to a boil and cook the potatoes for 5 minutes, then drain.

4. Boiling the diced potatoes in a pot of water.

5. Heat the oil in a large cast-iron or non-stick pan over medium heat. Add the potatoes to the pan and try to get them in a single, flat layer. Cook without stirring for about 4-5 minutes, so that the bottom gets nice and golden.

6. Sauteeing the potatoes in pan.

7. Add the green onion, and garlic, and stir for another 1-2 minutes.

8. Adding green onions and other ingredients to the pan.

9. Add the diced chicken, dried cranberries, thyme, salt, and pepper. Saute for another 5-10 minutes, or until the potatoes are soft and the turkey is warmed through.

10. Adding the turkey, cranberries, and seasonings to the pan.

11. You can serve the turkey cranberry hash as a side dish, or top it with an egg for a breakfast meal.

12. Plating an individual serving of turkey cranberry hash with a poached egg.

Prep Time: 5 Minutes

Cook Time: 25 Minutes

Servings: 4

Ingredients

- 4 pieces bacon
- 2 green onions, sliced, with green and white parts separated
- 1 tablespoon olive oil
- 4 large eggs
- 1/2 cup shredded cheddar cheese
- Salt and pepper
- 1/2 avocado, small diced
- 2 tablespoons chopped cilantro
- 4 tortillas

Instructions

1. Preheat your oven to 400F/200C. Place the bacon on a baking tray and bake for 18-20 minutes, or until crispy. Let dry on a paper towel.

2. Heat the olive oil in a pan on medium heat, add the the white parts of the green onion and saute for 1 minute.

3. Sauteeing green onions for breakfast tacos.

4. Whisk together the eggs in a bowl, then pour the beaten eggs in the pan. Use a spatula to move the eggs while they cook, flipping them a few times, until they're soft and pillowy yet cooked through.

5. Assemble the breakfast tacos by adding a portion of eggs to a tortilla. Top that with a sprinkle of the green parts of the green onion, several pieces of crumbled bacon, diced avocado, a sprinkle of cheddar cheese, and fresh cilantro. Season with salt and pepper.

6. A plate with two breakfast tacos.

Prep Time: 15 Minutes

Cook Time: 25 Minutes

Servings: 4

Ingredients

- 2 tablespoons extra-virgin olive oil
- 2 cups diced cooked corned beef
- 2 cups diced cooked potatoes (I'm using Yukon gold)
- 1 yellow onion, diced
- 1 green bell pepper, diced
- ½ teaspoon kosher salt
- ¼ teaspoon freshly ground black pepper
- 2 tablespoons roughly chopped fresh parsley
- Optional: poached eggs or fried eggs to top on the hash

Instructions

1. In a large cast-iron skillet, heat the olive oil over medium-high heat and add the onions and bell

pepper. Saute for 3 to 4 minutes, until the onion is translucent and softened.

2. Sauteing onions and pepper in a skillet for corned beef hash

3. Add the corned beef, and potatoes, and stir everything together. Then use a spatula to press down and flatten the ingredients in the pan. Cook for 3 to 4 minutes without stirring so that the bottom gets crispy and browned.

4. Cooking a corned beef hash in a black skillet

5. Use a spatula to flip the hash over and cook the other side for another couple of minutes. Stir in the parsley, salt, and pepper.

6. A skillet filled with corned beef hash

7. Enjoy plain or serve with poached eggs or fried eggs on top.

8. A plate filled with corned beef hash and an egg

11. Vegan Noodle with Vegetables

Prep Time: 15 Minutes

Cook Time: 20 Minutes

Servings: 4

Ingredients

- 1 small zucchini, seeds removed and cut into strips
- 1 small yellow squash, seeds removed and cut into strips
- ¼ teaspoon salt
- 2 instant ramen noodles (vegan) (use the noodles only and discard the sauce package)
- 1 tablespoon oil
- 8 ounces mushroom, sliced
- 2 tablespoon vegan butter, divided
- ¼ large onion, thinly sliced
- 2 tablespoons soy sauce
- 1 tablespoon vegetarian mushroom stir fry sauce
- Black pepper to taste

- Thinly sliced green onion and sesame seeds (for garnish)

Instructions

1. Remove the seeds of zucchini and yellow squash. Cut into thin strips lengthwise and cut into 2-inch pieces.
2. In a medium-size bowl, place a clean paper towel. Transfer the zucchini and yellow squash and sprinkle ¼ teaspoon of salt over them. Toss with your hands so the salt will even coat the zucchini and yellow squash. Set aside.
3. In a medium pot, boil water for instant ramen. Use the noodles only and discard the sauce package. Cook the ramen noodle 1 minute less than what it says in the instruction.
4. Drain and rinse the ramen noodle under cold water. Set aside.
5. On a large skillet, add 1 tablespoon of oil and cook the mushroom for a couple of minutes. Add a pinch of salt to help release the water from the mushroom.
6. Once the mushroom is wilted, add 1 tablespoon of butter and minced garlic. Cook with frequent stirring until it is fragrant, about 30-45 seconds.

7. Dap the water from the zucchini and yellow squash with a paper towel and add them to the pan with sliced onion.

8. Continue to cook for a minute or two.

9. Add the ramen noodle, soy sauce, and vegetarian mushroom stir fry sauce to the vegetable mix.

10. By using tongs, mix until everything is well coated with the sauce. Continue to cook for additional 2-3 minutes.

11. Remove the pan from the heat and add 1 tablespoon of butter. The heat from the noodle and vegetable should melt the butter.

12. Garnish with some black pepper, green onion, and sesame seeds. Serve right away.

Prep Time: 25 Minutes

Cook Time: 25 Minutes

Servings: 2

Ingredients

Sushi Rice:

- 3 cups cooked sushi rice (short grain rice)
- 1 tablespoon apple cider vinegar
- 1 tablespoon rice wine vinegar
- 1 tablespoon sugar
- ½ teaspoon salt
- Spicy Mayo Sauce:
- 3 tablespoons vegan mayo
- 1 tablespoon sweet chili sauce
- 1 tablespoon sriracha

Sushi Bowl:

- 4 to 6 vegan fishless filets, cooked according to package (I used Gardein's Golden Fishless Filet)
- ⅓ English cucumber, diced into small cubes
- 2 small avocados or 1 large avocado, diced

- 1 small green onion, thinly sliced (for garnish)

Instructions

1. Bake the vegan fishless filets according to their package.
2. While the fishless filets are baking, mix together apple cider vinegar, rice wine vinegar, sugar, and salt in a small bowl. Stir until sugar and salt are dissolved. Add the mixture to the cooked sushi rice. Set aside.
3. In another small bowl, mix together vegan mayo, sweet chili sauce, and sriracha. Set aside.
4. Assemble the sushi bowl. Place the seasoned sushi rice in a bowl, about 1 and ½ cups. Add the diced cucumber, vegan fishless filets, and avocado. Drizzle with vegan spicy mayo sauce. Garnish with green onion.

Prep Time: 10 Minutes

Cook Time: 10 Minutes

Servings: 6

Ingredients

- 6 sweet dinner roll, cut in half
- 4 tablespoons pesto of your choice
- 1 to 2 fresh mozzarella cheese balls, sliced
- 2 small tomatoes, sliced
- Salt and pepper to taste
- Red pepper flakes (optional)
- 2 to 3 tablespoons balsamic glaze

Instructions

1. Place the sliced mozzarella cheese on a clean kitchen towel or paper towel to absorb its access water.
2. Slice the dinner roll in half. Slice the tomato and set it aside.
3. Spread 1 teaspoon of pesto on the bottom of each roll.

4. Spread 1 teaspoon of pesto on the top part of each roll. Set them aside.

5. Place the sliced mozzarella cheese and tomato on the bottom of each roll.

6. Sprinkle with salt, pepper, and red pepper flakes.

7. Drizzle with balsamic glaze.

8. Top with the other half of the roll and serve right away.

Prep Time: 15 Minutes

Cook Time: 20 Minutes

Servings: 4

Ingredients

- 2 5-ounce cans tuna, drained
- 1 cup broccoli rice
- 1/3 cup mayonnaise
- 1/2 tablespoon Dijon mustard
- 2 green onions, sliced
- 2 tablespoons sunflower seeds
- 1-2 tablespoons chopped parsley, chives or other herbs
- salt and pepper, to taste

Instructions

1. Remove the florets from a head of broccoli, place in a food processor, and pulse until the texture resembles rice.

2. Broccoli being processed in a food processor for broccoli tuna salad.

3. Add the drained canned tuna, mayonnaise, dijon mustard, broccoli rice, sunflower seeds, green onion, and chopped parsley to a bowl.

4. Ingredients for broccoli tuna salad in a bowl.

5. Stir everything together until it's well combined.

6. Enjoy the broccoli tuna salad straight out of the bowl, turned into a sandwich, or wrapped in lettuce leaves.

Prep Time: 15 Minutes

Cook Time: 45 Minutes

Servings: 2

Ingredients

- 2 1/2 pound butternut squash
- 1 tablespoon avocado oil, or olive oil
- Salt and pepper, to taste
- 1/2 pound Italian sausage
- 1/2 onion, diced
- 3 garlic cloves, minced
- 2 cups (lightly packed) baby spinach
- 1 apple, diced
- 1 tablespoon fresh sage, finely chopped
- 1/2 tablespoon fresh rosemary, finely chopped
- 1/3 cup dried cranberries, unsweetened
- 1/4 cup pecans, chopped

Instructions

1. Preheat your oven to 400 degrees fahrenheit (200 degrees celsius).
2. Slice the butternut squash in half with a very sharp knife. You can also cut the ends off and microwave for 2 minutes, to make it easier to slice in half lengthwise.
3. Scoop the seeds out of the butternut squash with a spoon.
4. Lightly oil the butternut squash and season with salt and pepper.
5. Lay the butternut squash, cut side down on a baking sheet and bake for 40-45 minutes.
6. While the butternut squash is cooking, add the sausage to a saute pan on medium heat. Use a spatula to break up the sausage and cook until it's just browned.
7. Add the onions, garlic and baby spinach to the pan and stir for 2-3 minutes, or until the spinach is wilted.
8. Add the apple, sage and rosemary and cook for another 2-3 minutes, or until the apple has softened slightly.
9. Turn off the heat and stir in the cranberries and pecans.

10. When the butternut squash halves are cooked through, remove them from the oven, flip them over and remove some of the flesh (but leave plenty to enjoy!) to make room for the filling. Save this removed flesh and turn it into mashed butternut squash to enjoy later!

11. Fill the butternut squash with the apple sausage filling.

12. Turn the top broiler on the oven and bake the filled butternut squash for 5 minutes, or until they're golden on top. Serve immediately.

Prep Time: 10 Minutes

Cook Time: 1hrs 5 Minutes

Servings: 4

Ingredients

- 4 sweet potatoes
- 3 medium chicken breasts
- 2 tbsp avocado oil, or olive oil
- 3/4 cup chicken broth
- 8 ounces or more BBQ sauce
- 1/2 cup sliced red onion
- 1/3 cup chopped cilantro
- Salt and pepper, to taste

Instructions

1. Preheat your oven to 400 degrees fahrenheit.
2. Line a baking sheet with parchment paper and wash your sweet potatoes. Poke the sweet potatoes 5-6 times with a fork or sharp knife, place them on the baking sheet and bake for 60 minutes. If you have

large or small sweet potatoes you may need to adjust the bake time.

3. While the sweet potatoes are baking, drizzle the oil in a sauté pan on medium heat. Add the chicken breasts, season with salt and pepper and cook for 5 minutes. Flip the chicken over, add the chicken broth, cover the pan and cook for an additional 7-10 minutes or until the chicken is cooked through (to 165 degrees fahrenheit). Remove the chicken from pan and shred with two forks or a stand mixer (see my Shredded Chicken post for more details).

4. Add the shredded chicken to a bowl and mix with the BBQ sauce.

5. Slice each sweet potato in half, fill with BBQ chicken and top with red onion and cilantro.

Prep Time: 10 Minutes

Cook Time: 15 Minutes

Servings: 4

Ingredients

For The Chicken:

- 150g / 5oz cooked chicken
- 1/2 tsp oregano
- 1/2 tsp chili powder
- 1 tsp paprika
- 1 tbsp lemon juice
- 1 tsp olive oil
- 1/4 cup chopped parsley
- black pepper
- 2 garlic cloves
- 1/2 pointed red pepper

Salad:

- 1/4 avocado
- 1 cucumber
- 1 tomato

- 4-5 basil leaves
- 3 radishes
- 1/3 red onion
- 1 tsp olive oil
- salt and pepper

Additionally:

- Feta
- Olives

Instructions

1. Shred the chicken and add it with the pointed red pepper to a nonstick pan with a little bit of olive oil. Stir in the oregano, paprika, black pepper, chili powder and garlic. Stir for about 2-3 minutes, add in the lemon juice and take off heat. Stir through the parsley.
2. Add all ingredients for the salad to a bowl, toss together.
3. Place the chicken on one side of a serving bowl, the salad on another, then add the feta cheese on top and some olives on the side.

4. You can also serve these bowls with some delicious yogurt garlic sauce made by mixing 2/3 cup yogurt with salt and 1-2 minced cloves of garlic.
5. Serve immediately and enjoy!

Prep Time: 10 Minutes

Cook Time: 15 Minutes

Servings: 4

Ingredients

- 1/2 sweet potato, chopped (around 200g)
- 2 cups chopped potatoes
- 12oz/350g ground turkey
- 1 onion, chopped
- 2 garlic cloves, minced
- 1 tsp mint, dried
- 1 tsp cumin
- 1 tbsp oil
- 1 ½ tbsp tomato paste
- 1 tsp paprika
- 1 1/3 cup water to cover
- 2 tbsp chopped parsley

Instructions

1. Chop the potatoes, and the onion and mince the garlic.

2. Add the onion, garlic and ground turkey to the skillet with a little bit of olive oil and stir at medium heat for 2-3 minutes.

3. Add in the chopped potatoes, sweet potatoes, salt and black pepper, tomato paste, paprika, cumin and mint. Stir well and cover with water (about a cup).

4. Cover the skillet with a lid and let simmer at a lower temperature for about 30 minutes.

5. After 30 minutes the potatoes should be done and your moussaka is ready to serve!

6. Sprinkle some thinly chopped parsley all over and serve with some salad and yogurt-based garlic sauce as described or with this cashew sauce if you're dairy-free.

Prep Time: 10 Minutes

Cook Time: 20 Minutes

Servings: 4

Ingredients

- ¼ cup raw cashew
- ½ cup unsweetened almond milk
- 1 tablespoon oil
- 1 tablespoon vegan butter (or use another tablespoon of oil)
- ½ large onion, diced
- 2 teaspoons ginger, minced or grated
- 3 cloves garlic, minced
- 1 teaspoon cumin
- 1 teaspoon garam masala (I like this brand)
- ½ tablespoon curry powder
- ¼ teaspoon turmeric powder
- ½ teaspoon paprika
- ¼ teaspoon ground black pepper
- 3 tablespoons tomato paste
- 1 cup cauliflower floret

- 1 cup diced potato
- 2-3 small size carrots, cut into small pieces
- ½ teaspoon salt
- 1 cup water (or vegetable broth)
- 2 teaspoons Vegan Chicken Flavor Bouillon Powder (omit if using vegetable broth)
- ½ cup frozen peas

Rice and/or naan for serving

Instructions

1. In a high-speed blender, blend together cashew and almond milk until smooth. Set aside.
2. In a large non-stick skillet, heat oil and butter together and add diced onion. Cook until onion becomes translucent.
3. Add the minced garlic and ginger. Cook until fragrant, about a minute.
4. Add tomato paste, cumin, garam masala, curry powder, turmeric, paprika, and black pepper. Stir until everything is well mixed and bubbles a little in the pan.

5. Add cauliflower carrot, potato, water, and vegan chicken flavor bouillon powder (or vegetable broth). Add the salt.

6. Bring the mixture to a boil and place a lid on top. Reduce the heat to medium and continue to cook for 5-7 minutes until the potato is cooked but not mushy.

7. Add the cashew almond milk mixture and frozen pea to the curry. Stir to mix and continue to cook for additional 2-3 minutes.

8. Serve hot with rice and/or naan.

Prep Time: 10 Minutes

Cook Time: 20 Minutes

Servings: 4

Ingredients

Burger Patties:

- 1 can black beans, rinsed and drained
- 1 tbsp hot paprika
- 1/2 tbsp crushed red pepper
- 1 tsp black pepper
- 1 tsp cumin
- 3 garlic cloves
- 2 mushrooms, chopped
- ½ onion, grated
- 1 tbsp flax meal
- salt
- 2 tbsp greens
- 1 tbsp sesame seeds

Additionally:

- buns

- jalapeno

- mustard

- tomato paste

- onion

Instructions

1. Sauté the mushrooms with some salt and olive oil in a non-stick pan.

2. Prepare all ingredients that will go into the burger patties - grate the onion, rinse and drain the canned black beans, peel and mince the garlic, chop the greens (I had some leftover kale, basil and parsley).

3. Add all ingredients for the burger patties to a bowl, add salt and start mashing it all together using a fork. You want a mixture that sticks together, but is still quite chunky.

4. Form patties and fry them in a nonstick pan with some olive oil on both sides until nicely brown.

5. Assemble your burgers with the ingredients you like (I toasted the buns, used tomato paste, because I hate ketchup, some onions, some mustard, some jalapeno and a tomato - it was delicious!).

6. Enjoy!

21. Super Fresh Corn and Avocado Salad

Prep Time: 10 Minutes

Cook Time: 15 Minutes

Servings: 3

Ingredients

- 1 avocado, chopped
- 1/2 corn on the cob
- 2 cups lettuce
- 2 tomatoes, chopped
- 1 cucumber, chopped
- 1 zucchini, sliced & grilled
- 1/3 cup olives
- 1/2 red onion, small, chopped
- bunch parsley
- 1 garlic clove, minced
- 1 Tbsp olive oil
- 1/4 cup crumbled feta cheese
- 1/2 lemon, juice of
- flax seeds or sesame seeds

- salt and pepper to taste

Instructions

1. Wash, slice and cook the zucchini or saute it in a pan with some olive oil.
2. Boil the corn and cut the kernels off.
3. Chop lettuce, tomato, onion, cucumber, parsley, avocado.
4. Add the vegetables to a salad bowl.
5. Mince the garlic, juice the lemon and add them to that bowl.
6. Once cooled off, add in the grilled zucchini and the corn.
7. Sprinkle some olive oil and feta cheese and toss to combine.
8. Have a taste and add salt and pepper to taste. Sprinkle flax seeds or toasted sesame seeds for even more flavor.
9. Serve immediately!

Prep Time: 10 Minutes

Cook Time: 30 Minutes

Servings: 6

Ingredients

- 1 ½ pounds boneless, skinless chicken thighs
- ½ cup full fat Greek yogurt
- 1 tablespoon fresh lemon juice
- 2 teaspoons minced ginger
- 3 garlic cloves, minced
- 1 teaspoon Kashmiri red chili powder
- 1 teaspoon garam masala
- 1 teaspoon ground turmeric
- 1 teaspoon salt
- 2 tablespoons extra-virgin olive oil or avocado oil

For The Butter Sauce:

- 1 medium yellow onion, diced
- 2 teaspoons minced ginger
- 3 garlic cloves, minced
- 1 teaspoon Kashmiri red chili powder

- 1 teaspoon garam masala
- ½ teaspoon ground coriander
- ½ teaspoon cumin
- ¼ cup raw cashews
- 1 tablespoon coconut sugar (or other sweetener)
- 1 (15-ounce) can crushed tomatoes
- 1 cup water
- 2 tablespoons unsalted butter (or ghee)
- ½ cup heavy cream (or coconut cream)

For Serving:

- basmatic rice
- freshly chopped cilantro

Instructions

1. Dice the chicken. Cut the chicken into 1-inch pieces and place it in a bowl.
2. Diced chicken in a bowl for butter chicken
3. Marinate the chicken. Add the yogurt, lemon juice, ginger, garlic, red chili powder, garam masala, turmeric, and salt to the bowl. Stir it all together, then cover and refrigerate for an hour (or up to overnight).
4. Marinated chicken in a glass bowl for butter chicken

5. Cook the chicken. Heat the oil over medium-high heat in a large saute pan. Place the marinated chicken in the fry pan and cook for 5 to 6 minutes, until the chicken is opaque. Transfer the chicken to a separate bowl.

6. Cooked chicken pieces in a pan for butter chicken

7. Make the sauce. Add the onions to the pan and saute for 3 to 4 minutes, until softened and translucent.

8. A pan with cooked onions for butter chicken

9. Add the ginger, garlic, red chili powder, garam masala, coriander, cumin, and stir for another minute. Then add the cashews, crushed tomatoes, sugar, and water. Stir it all together, reduce the heat to low, and simmer for 5 minutes.

10. Butter chicken curry sauce in a large pan with spoon.

11. Transfer the sauce to a high-powered blender and blend for a minute, until smooth and creamy.

12. Blending butter chicken curry sauce in a blender

13. Combine it all together. Wipe the pan clean with a paper towel (if you'd like to remove any lumps from the final sauce), then stir together the creamy butter sauce, butter, and heavy cream.

14. Making butter chicken curry sauce in a large pan

15. Add the chicken back to the pan over medium heat and stir with the sauce for 3 to 5 minutes, until the chicken is warmed and cooked through.

16. A large skillet with butter chicken

17. To serve. Enjoy the butter chicken on it's own, or serve it over basmati rice topped with fresh cilantro.

Prep Time: 15 Minutes

Cook Time: 30 Minutes

Servings: 5

Ingredients

- 2 tablespoons extra-virgin olive oil
- 3 large leeks
- 2 garlic cloves, minced
- 4 cups vegetable broth, or more for a thinner texture
- 2 pounds Yukon Gold potatoes, peeled and diced into ½-inch pieces
- 1 teaspoon kosher salt
- 1 bay leaf
- 2 sprigs of fresh thyme
- freshly chopped chives and black pepper for garnish

Instructions

1. Slice the stem and green leaves off the leeks, leaving the white and light green parts. Cut the leeks in half lengthwise, then chop across.

2. Chopped leeks on a wooden cutting board

3. Place the chopped leeks into a colander and run under cold water to remove dirt and debris.

4. Chopped leeks in a colander for potato leek soup

5. Heat the olive oil in a large pot or Dutch oven over medium heat. Add the leeks and sauté for 8 to 10 minutes, until softened (but not browned). Then add the garlic and stir for another minute.

6. Sauteing leeks in a pot for

7. Add the diced potatoes, salt, bay leaf, thyme, and vegetable stock. Increase the heat to high and bring to a boil, then reduce the heat to low, cover, and simmer for 15 to 20 minutes, until the potatoes are fork tender.

8. Cooking potato leek soup in a white pot

9. Remove and discard the bay leaf and thyme sprigs. Use an immersion blender to blend the soup until your desired level of creaminess. Alternatively, you can blend the soup in batches in a high-powered blender.

10. A bowl of creamy potato leek soup

11. Top the potato leek soup with chopped chives and freshly ground black pepper before serving.

Prep Time: 15 Minutes

Cook Time: 7hrs 30 Minutes

Servings: 6

Ingredients

- 2 tablespoons avocado oil,
- 3 ½ pounds beef chuck roast
- 2 teaspoon salt
- 1 teaspoon freshly ground black pepper
- 4 cloves garlic, thinly sliced
- 1 yellow onion, cut into large chunks
- 4 carrots, peeled and cut into 1-inch pieces
- 3 stalks celery, cut into 1-inch pieces
- 1 ½ pounds baby potatoes (white or yukon gold), quartered
- 2 cups low-sodium beef broth
- 1 cup red wine,
- 2 sprigs fresh rosemary
- 2 sprigs fresh thyme
- 2 bay leaves

Optional To Thicken Gravy:

- 2 tablespoons arrowroot powder
- 3 tablespoons water

Instructions

1. In a large cast iron skillet, heat the oil on medium-high heat. Season both sides of the beef roast with salt and pepper, and sear for 4 to 5 minutes on each side to give it a dark brown crust. Transfer the roast to a 6 to 7-quart slow cooker.
2. Cooking beef in a skillet for slow cooker pot roast
3. Add the garlic, onion, carrots, celery, potatoes, rosemary, thyme, and bay leaves to the slow cooker. Pour the beef broth and red wine on top. Add the lid and cook on low for 8 to 9 hours or on high for 5 to 6 hours.
4. Adding potatoes into a slow cooker for pot roast
5. Remove the sprigs of rosemary, thyme, and the bay leaves. Then remove the roast and shred or slice it up.
6. A slow cooker with pot roast and herbs
7. If you'd like to thicken the broth to more of a gravy consistency, stir together the arrowroot powder and

water in a small bowl. Pour it into the slow cooker and stir everything together until it starts to thicken.

8. Pouring arrowroot mixture into slow cooker pot roast

9. Serve the meat and vegetables on a platter with some of the gravy (you can serve extra gravy on the side)

Prep Time: 15 Minutes

Cook Time: 45 Minutes

Servings: 6

Ingredients

- 1 ½ pound coho salmon (sockeye and king salmon also work)
- 3 tablespoons extra-virgin olive oil
- 1 orange
- 1 fennel bulb, halved and thinly sliced, reserving some fronds
- 1 shallot, thinly sliced
- ½ lemon, zested and juiced
- 2 teaspoons honey
- ½ cup chopped fresh herbs (basil, tarragon, dill, or mint)
- ½ teaspoon kosher salt
- ¼ teaspoon freshly cracked black pepper

Instructions

1. Preheat the oven to 200°F (93°C), and set a rack in the middle of the oven. Place the salmon on a parchment-lined baking sheet (skin side down), then brush the top with ½ tablespoon olive oil.

2. Slice the orange in half and juice one half, then peel the other half and thinly slice the fruit into half moons.

3. Sliced fresh oranges on a wooden board.

4. In a medium bowl, add the remaining 2 ½ tablespoons of olive oil, sliced fennel, orange pieces and juice, shallot, lemon zest and juice, honey, herbs, salt, and pepper. You can also add some fennel fronds if you'd like. Gently stir to combine.

5. Mixing fennel orange mixture in a bowl for slow roasted salmon

6. Add the orange fennel mixture to the top of the salmon. Roast the salmon for 30-45 minutes, depending on the thickness of the fish and how "done" you like it. I prefer the edges to be more "well done" and the center more "medium" (about 125°F/52°C). Note that the color will remain more vibrant orange than other baked salmon recipes, looking under-cooked, though it's not.

7. A sheet pan with slow roasted

8. Remove the salmon from the oven, serve it straight from the sheet pan and scoop any extra pan juices on top.

Prep Time: 15 Minutes

Cook Time: 15 Minutes

Servings: 6

Ingredients

- 6 pieces bacon, cut into 1-inch pieces
- 1 small onion, diced
- 3 cloves garlic, minced
- 2 tablespoons stone ground mustard, or Dijon mustard
- 1/4 teaspoon smoked paprika
- 1 head cabbage, sliced and chopped
- salt and pepper, to taste

Instructions

1. Heat a large pan on medium heat and add the sliced bacon. Cook until crispy, then removed to a paper towel lined plate.
2. Cooking bacon pieces in a pan.

3. Add the onion and saute for 2-3 minutes, or until it's translucent.

4. Add the garlic, mustard, smoked paprika, salt and pepper and give it a stir to combine. Then place the sliced cabbage on top and use a large spoon or tongs to stir and saute together for another 12-15 minutes.

5. Fried cabbage in a pan on the stove.

6. When the cabbage is done it should be soft and starting to caramelize. Then toss the bacon back in together.

Prep Time: 20 Minutes

Cook Time: 45 Minutes

Servings: 5

Ingredients

Chicken:

- 5 chicken thighs, skin-on and bone-in
- 2 tablespoons olive oil

Marinade:

- 2 lemons, juiced and zested (approx 1/4 cup of juice)
- 2 teaspoons Dijon Mustard
- 3 garlic cloves, minced
- 1 teaspoon dried oregano
- 1 teaspoon dried thyme
- 1/2 tsp salt
- 1/4 tsp black pepper
- 1 tablespoon olive oil

Rice:

1. 1 yellow onion, diced

2. 2 cups baby spinach, lightly packed and roughly chopped
3. 2 garlic cloves, minced
4. 1 teaspoons dried oregano
5. 1 cup long grain white rice
6. 2 cups chicken stock
7. 1/2 teaspoon salt
8. 1/4 teaspoon black pepper
9. chopped parsley, for garnish
10. lemon zest or slices, for garnish

Instructions

Marinate The Chicken:

1. Add all of the marinade ingredients to a bowl and stir together.
2. Making the chicken marinade.
3. Place chicken thighs in a glass dish, pour marinade over the chicken, and turn each piece to coat. Cover dish and marinate chicken in the fridge for at least 30 minutes and up to overnight.
4. Pouring the marinade on top of chicken thighs.

Cook The Chicken And Rice:

1. Preheat your oven to 350 degrees fahrenheit. In a large ovenproof skillet, heat 2 tablespoons olive oil on medium-high heat. Add chicken thighs skin-side down and cook until skin is golden brown, about 5 minutes. Reserve the leftover marinade as you'll add that back in later.

2. Searing the chicken skin side down in a pan.

3. Flip the chicken and cook another 5 minutes. Remove chicken thighs from skillet and set aside.

4. Use your tongs to scrape and remove any browned bits, and bunch up a couple of paper towels to soak up some fat from the pan, but not all. Reserve a little bit of grease to cook the onions.

5. Add the diced onions and stir for 1-2 minutes, or until they start to become translucent.

6. Adding the diced onions to the pan.

7. Add the chopped spinach, garlic, oregano, salt, pepper, and reserved marinade. Stir for another 30 seconds or until the spinach starts to wilt.

8. Add the rice to the skillet, and stir well to coat the rice with the oil.

9. Pour the chicken stock into the skillet and stir well. Bring this to a simmer on the stove.

10. Adding the chicken stock to the rice and other ingredients.

11. Arrange chicken thighs on top of the rice, then cover the skillet and place in the preheated oven. Bake for 35 minutes. Remove the lid, return the skillet to the oven, and bake until chicken is cooked through and rice is tender, about 10 minutes more.

12. Adding the chicken thighs on top of the rice, then placing the lid on top.

13. Let the chicken and rice rest for 5 to 10 minutes. The rice will look really dark as the spinach and onions rise to the surface. Just fluff the rice up with a fork to mix everything back together before serving.

14. Fluffing the rice in the pan with a fork.

15. Top with chopped parsley and grilled lemon slices or fresh lemon zest.

Prep Time: 15 Minutes

Cook Time: 20 Minutes

Servings: 4

Ingredients

- 2 pounds carrots, peeled
- 1/4 cup honey
- 3 garlic cloves, minced
- 2 tablespoons melted butter or ghee
- 1 tablespoon olive oil
- 1 teaspoon cinnamon
- 1/2 teaspoon ground ginger
- 1/2 teaspoon salt
- 1/4 teaspoon pepper
- parsley, thyme or other herbs for garnish (optional)

Instructions

1. Preheat your oven to 425F/220C. Then, cut the carrots on a diagonal, about 1"-1.5" in length. If your

carrots are large and thick, you can slice them in half as well.

2. Carrots being chopped for honey glazed carrots.

3. In a mixing bowl, toss the sliced carrots with the honey, garlic, butter, oil, and spices.

4. Honey glazed carrots being tossed in a glass bowl.

5. Pour the carrots and glaze onto a sheet pan and spread them out.

6. Honey glazed carrots on a sheet pan before baking.

7. Roast for 20-25 minutes, tossing halfway through. You can also broil for 2-3 minutes, to get caramelization on the edges.

8. Transfer carrots to a serving dish and garnish with chopped herbs.

Prep Time: 30 Minutes

Cook Time: 25 Minutes

Servings: 6

Ingredients

Marinade:

- 1/4 cup olive oil
- 2 tablespoons red wine vinegar
- 3 tablespoons lemon juice
- 1 teaspoon Dijon mustard
- 3 garlic cloves, minced
- 1 teaspoon dried oregano
- 1/2 teaspoon salt
- 1/4 teaspoon black pepper

Chicken Kabobs

- 1 1/2 pounds boneless skinless chicken breasts, about 3 large chicken breasts, cut into 1 1/2-inch pieces.
- 1 red bell pepper, seeded, cut into 1 1/2-Inch pieces
- 1 yellow bell pepper, seeded, cut into 1 1/2-inch pieces
- 1 red onion, cut into 1 1/2-inch chunks

- 1 zucchini, sliced

Instructions

1. To make the marinade, whisk together the olive oil, red wine vinegar, lemon juice, Dijon mustard, minced garlic, dried oregano, salt, and pepper.
2. Place chicken pieces in a glass dish and pour the marinade over the chicken. Cover and marinate in the fridge for at least one hour.
3. Light a gas or charcoal grill on medium-high heat. Thread the skewers with pieces of red onion, chicken, zucchini, and bell pepper. You can alternate the order.
4. Place the kabobs on the preheated grill, and cook about 5-7 minutes per side. The kabobs are done when the chicken is cooked through and the vegetables are lightly charred, about 15 minutes.
5. Serve with lemon wedges and tzatziki sauce.
6. Greek chicken kabobs with lemon wedges on a plate.

Prep Time: 10 Minutes

Cook Time: 10 Minutes

Servings: 2

Ingredients

Salmon Avocado Salad:

- 4 cups baby spinach
- 2 tomatoes, chopped
- 1 avocado, diced
- 1 cucumber, peeled and sliced
- 1/4 cup red onion, chopped
- 2 tablespoon olive oil
- 2 salmon filets
- salt and pepper, to taste

Dressing:

- 1 recipe lemon vinaigrette

Instructions

1. Heat olive oil in a large pan over medium-high heat. Season the salmon filets with salt and pepper. Add the salmon filets top side down and cook for 4-5 minutes.

2. Flip the salmon and cook for an additional 2-3 minutes or until the salmon is mostly opaque, with just a smidge of softness still in the middle.

3. Divide all of the other salad ingredients between two bowls, then place the cooked salmon on top.

4. Mix the dressing ingredients together in a small bowl and drizzle on top.